About Jessica Sutter

Jessica is a homeschooling, entrepreneur, mama to four precocious, change maker buddhas (cause they are her teachers every freakin' day...) who is lit up by supporting people to heal and integrate those parts of themselves who've been lost or are yet hidden and then to create the beautiful life their heart and soul are calling them to.

She has been on her own conscious, breathtaking journey for 13 years. She's read mountains of books and worked with amazing teachers, healers, mentors, and coaches. In addition to having a gift for empathic and intuitive healing, Jessica has lots of useful skills, information, gifts, and talents to share.

It has been her experience that those around us arc mirrors; they show us just what we need to see to do our precious work of reclaiming our life. This can make life and relationships messy and beautiful all at the same time and is a priceless tool.

Jessica's work is all about you and supporting you in being the you, you feel your heart and soul calling you to be; the one aching to be shared and seen.

You've got a sixth sense about this life and your mission here and it feels BIG. You've got big responsibilities (You may have littles that came here to get some shit done too!), desires (OH MY), plans, and some pretty breathtaking demons that seem to hold you back. Yes?

Jessica has SO been there, Love. So.

You're in just the right place. Jessica would love to work with you to support you in your own great work, and in living your life on purpose. To connect, visit her website at www.JessicaSutter.com or email at jessicasutterconnect@gmail.com.

Introduction

So. What is Metabolism?

You've heard this word before. We use it in our culture to describe our digestion and how quickly, easily, or slowly our bodies 'deal' with the food we put into them.

 I invite you to consider an alternative, and perhaps more accurate, definition as it will be used in this book. Metabolism, as your fire; that which keeps you at your healthiest.

A person with a healthy metabolism is happy, strong, has good digestion and immunity, a normal bodily temperature of AT LEAST 98 degrees, feels warm and comfortable (no cold hands/feet; yes EVEN in the winter!), sleeps peacefully through the night without waking to use the bathroom, has a lack of premenstrual symptoms (if you are a woman ;)), there is a 'glow' about them and their life. These are just a few of the 'symptoms' of a person with a truly healthy metabolism.

The way in which one goes about maintaining a healthy metabolism, or revitalizing one that is low, is *highly* individual. I believe this is supremely excellent and magical news! There is much more involved here than simply eating well, exercising, and getting proper rest.

YOU are more than a body. You are a WHOLE BEING with a body, mind, spirit, and soul. You are a magnificently unique *individual*. What works for your friends or family *may not* work for you, and vice versa, at any given moment in time. In the pages that follow, you will be introduced to a variety of ways to maintain, strengthen, or heal your metabolism to live the most vibrant life possible.

Metabolism, Nutrition, and You...

A Heartfelt Introductory Guide to Creating the Most Magnificent Vehicle for Your Spirit and Soul to Travel This Earthly Journey

I began this project to create a nutritional e-book that would contain simple information and science about nutrition you most likely have not encountered before, but life changing to be sure...

You see, this information is not mainstream and I find 'different' fascinating. It speaks to my soul.

In researching and writing this information I found I became stuck. Stuck, Stuck, STUCK!!! And then I realized I was stuck because I wasn't speaking from my heart, my truth. Our health is SO much more than just keeping our bodies well.... AND....

I don't hold all the answers for this. The information shared here can be true at any time, or not at all. I was frustrated because I don't have *one* answer. But the truth is... there isn't *one* answer for the world's woes. The world is made up of many people, each unique, and yet the same. So many pieces go into the creation of our personal Masterpieces; our Beings.

And really, we all hold our own truth and answers to our own healing.

Our health, as we have been led to believe by mainstream 'medicine', is NOT comprised of simply our body. There is NOT a very simple answer to the frustrating state of our health. So many things have happened and gone into the demise of our health. Much has become unbalanced.

It is not just the food we eat, or the state of busyness and stress we maintain. It is not just pesticides, drugs, vaccines, poisonous ingredients in our cleaning and beauty products, etc. *It is all of these things; and more.*

What can *I* offer you?

I can offer you hope and empowerment.

These feel like the most beautiful thing I can offer right now. I can share with you things I know to be true; at least for myself. I can share with you suggestions and ideas and intuition about what may be happening and what may work for you based on what I've learned over the last 11 years (at the time of this writing). Ultimately, and really, it is up to you.

Our beings are made up of a body, mind, spirit, and soul and each of these needs to be in alignment with the other, and our own personal truth, in order for us to be ultimately and truly healthy.

AND as the ultimate goal and purpose of humanity is to *grow and become more of who we are,* each of these aspects of self are going to be in an almost constant process of change and growth. So, our health can potentially be in constant change because our being is working to maintain balance. This doesn't have to be a battle or struggle, however.

Our physical health is largely effected by our emotional and spiritual health and also by the sorts of earthly good or toxic things with which we nourish ourselves.

Our physical symptoms are a big clue to our emotional and spiritual issues. This has been repeatedly true for me and research has substantiated this point. If you are curious you could do an internet search for Louise L. Hay, Dr. Bruce Lipton, or Dr. Bradley Nelson or try 'Do our emotions effect our physical health?' You are bright and intelligent and I am certain you will find what you are searching for.

And so, with that said, here is the advice I can share with you about your whole health.

The word 'nourish' feels really whole and deeply good to me when I think of health, and feeling and being healthy, so I am using it to help share these ideas with you.

Nourish your body with food that is as close to the earth and free of pesticides and processing as you can find, grow, and/or afford. (I once listened to an incredibly informative and inspirational TED talk by an 11 year old boy who said, "You can pay the farmer or you can pay the doctor." *Bloody Brilliant*.) Pesticides have been very directly linked to MANY diseases such as Alzheimer's and cancer.

Look as closely as what grows naturally (including what we've been taught are weeds!) in your own backyard; as long as you know there are no pesticides in your yard.

Some examples of things you'd look for are lamb's quarters, plantain (yes, these are ALSO bananas) sheep sorrel, wood sorrel, violets, chickweed, clover, purslane. If your grass is dying, from drought for instance, and you still have some 'weeds' growing...look them up. They are there for a purpose. There is a magical reason they are surviving when your grass is not. They are there to replenish the earth, and *you*.

These plants are a tremendous source of nutrition for, first your soil, which allows whatever plants are growing in it to absorb these nutrients and goodness, and thus pass it along to animals who eat it, and you...Food Web Baby!

The greens that grow wild in your yard contain crazy amounts of nutrients. Nettles (which you can eat once dried or boiled) or lamb's quarters, for instance, contain more calcium ounce per ounce than milk, and are easier to digest. Each of the herbs mentioned above also have amazing healing properties. Violets and plantain are both excellent expectorants; violets for dry congestion and plantain for wet. Doing an internet search on these miracles will yield you a rich list of information on their healing properties!

Your body wants, and needs mostly plants, in the form of root vegetables such as potatoes, carrots, sweet potatoes, yams, carrots, turnips, rutabagas, and beets for example. You also need other vegetables and fruits, as fresh and unaltered as possible. As a mammal with canine teeth your body DOES need some meat. It provides the source of vitamin B12 your body needs for making blood cells and maintaining a healthy nervous system among other things. If you do not feel okay about eating meat however, there are plant based alternatives and I would recommend consuming them.

Forcing ourselves to consume or do anything we do not feel good about, has great potential to cause great unbalance and detriment to our health. *Follow your heart in all matters*. Also remember, just because others do something you do not agree with does not mean they are wrong. They simply do things *differently* than you. I know this is difficult to digest (sorry about the pun.). I am finding it more true all the time.

Grains. I know there is great hype about gluten free grains and even no grains at all. I tried this for three years and ended up more unhealthy and miserable than I was when I started. I believe I took it too far for too long and became a bit of a zealot, if you will, about food. I've been around the block, and further, with food. It is where my journey of healing from postpartum depression began. I found I ended up more lost and with more questions with each new idea I tried. At this point, I feel most happy, healthy, and comfortable following what my body is asking for and eating a good variety of foods. When we eat the same thing for too long, we get issues. Remember...we are creatures of habit, and who change often to maintain balance and for growth.

There are many grains in the world. Spelt, rice, barley, quinoa, amaranth, and millet, for example. I'd invite you to give them a try. It will change up your diet and introduce a new flavor and new meal ideas which is always a delightful idea. They also have awesome nutrients, especially B vitamins which are great for helping keeping stress levels lower.

Many of these grains are also ground into flour and can be baked with, and are even made into, noodles. Your recipes may need to be tweaked a bit to make them work right. Doing a simple internet search for baking with the particular flour you are using will be helpful. I spent 3 years modifying my baking recipes to fit my diet. It was a change, but not crazy difficult. Stores now also sell premixed flours for baking.

Grains fall into the category of carbohydrates as do vegetables and fruits and sugars. Our bodies use carbohydrates as fuel. Fuel is necessary to keep fires burning at their optimal level and so consuming them as a large portion of our diet is beneficial, contrary to popular opinion. For more information, I direct you to www.180degreehealth.com

Wheat has become a demon in our society. Thousands of years ago wheat was different. It has been changed over time and is not the same 'creature' it was initially and so does not work in our systems the same way...though really, we eat a lot of it and it is highly processed (foods that are processed are not digested in our bodies the same way as unprocessed and also do not contain the same number of nutrients the food originally had. This can cause digestive issues and allergies or food intolerances, over time.). When we eat a bun with our burgers and bread with our sandwiches and toast with our breakfast and noodles with our sauce, they are all made out of wheat. So adding or changing this up, just a little bit, by using a different type (not brand) of flour or purchasing some spelt noodles, for instance, could make a beautiful difference in your diet.

Your body needs a harmonious balance of **salt** and **sugar**. Your taste buds will literally tell you what that harmonious balance is for you and this will change very often. Remember your body was beautifully and magnificently created to maintain health and heal when needed. One amazing way it tells you what it needs is through your satiety signals; taste buds AND that beautiful *sigh* you emit after you'd had a satisfying meal where you feel all full and content.

Table sugar or salt are okay sometimes. They are also processed and so are stripped of lovely nutrients your body needs. Sea salt is great for nutrients and taste. It does cost more. I consider it an investment in my health and that of my family. Remember the farmer or the doctor!

Here are some sugar alternatives for those times when you'd like to change things up a bit...maple syrup, honey (Honey is incredible when it is raw. Whole books have been written on the benefits and beauty of honey! It is liquid gold!) turbinado sugar, rapadura, blackstrap molasses (which is beautifully high in iron pregnant mamas!)There are others you could find including molasses and fruit.

I recommend exercising caution about corn syrup, especially high fructose corn syrup and even stevia. (This is an herb, and so, when used in its natural form, a *green* plant, is lovely. The *white* powder sold in stores means the stevia has been processed, altered from its natural form,

13

and could cause issues.) Both are highly processed and this processing is something our bodies are not always sure what to do with. On the other hand, there are times when eating highly processed foods can help us on our road back to health. For more information on this I highly recommend checking out www.180degreehealth.com. There are some amazing folks there and I have personally worked with Matt Stone. This guy knows his stuff and is lots of fun! He has also gathered other amazing people who know their stuff and are equally fun! Like attracts like afterall.

Fat is also incredibly important for your body. However, you want to provide your body with safe and healthy fats. Our bodies need sufficient amounts of good quality *saturated* fats like coconut oil, butter, and beef tallow to keep our systems running smoothly and for nutrient absorption.

I know what we've been taught about saturated fats. AND it is *GREAT* to question well, EVERYTHING!

My family has a history of heart disease and cancer and yet, because of the research I've done and information I now understand, I choose to eat a more traditional diet containing saturated fats, mostly coconut oil and butter, and occasionally olive oil.

I choose this because other fats are far too aggravating and grating on our system. They cause free radicals and inflammation like crazy. *Inflammation is the cause of most*

14

every disease known to humanity. For more information on this I, again, highly recommend looking into the work of Matt Stone, and others, of www.180degreehealth.com.

I also choose this because saturated fat creates a beautiful blanket, if you will, over nerves and other precious places in our bodies. This is important for our children as they are growing and learning and for us and our children as we are attempting to stay calm and out of stress and anxiety. It allows for smooth flow of information in our brains and nervous system as well as veins and arteries. Think of a bumpy, torn up road vs. a brand new, smooth road. Got it???

Dairy can be a tricky thing also. If you have trouble tolerating it, I'd invite you to take a break from it for a while, perhaps about a month, and then slowly reintroduce it. If you truly cannot tolerate it there are substitutes you can use for milk in recipes. I found almond milk to be heavenly and creamy and very easy to make. There is also rice milk and soy. Soy is a whole other subject and I invite you to look up some serious pros and cons of soy. I personally stay away from it as much as possible.

To make almond milk, you will need to soak almonds in water in a covered bowl for about 12 hours. You then blend them in a blender with new water and strain the 'milk'. Done. Enjoy!!

Ultimately, where food and nutrition is concerned, FOLLOW YOUR CRAVINGS!!! Your body was magnificently and magically created to KNOW what it needs; what YOU need. I know it seems counterintuitive if your body is craving sugar like mad, *AND* there is a built in starvation mechanism, if you will, that gets triggered when we live our lives from a place of lack or not enough. Sugar is fast energy and helps your body store fat. Why is this a GOOD thing you may be wondering??? It is a GOOD thing because, when your body goes into starvation mode, the surest and easiest way to get it OUT of starvation mode and to begin LOSING weight is to give it what it is craving so that it realizes there is no longer a LACK of anything and it doesn't NEED to store up 'resources' aka: fat anymore. At this point, there is potential for your body to begin to burn fat spontaneously.

There is, again, FANTASTIC information on this phenomenon over at www.180degreehealth.com!!! There is awesome research available to read!

Sugar also helps you when you are under stress and/or feeling sad or unhappy. If this is going on for an extended period of time, there is something deeper that is calling out to you to be addressed and I'd invite you to seek out help. AND, I'd also invite you to lean into, to *trust*, what your body is asking for. Feed it all it wants until it wants NO MORE and then check in and see what it is asking for next and follow that. This just might lead you to the most glorious discoveries!!!

Patience, a good year, is a virtue when raising your metabolism and regaining your health. As are some, perhaps somewhat unpleasant 'side effects' such as gradual weight gain (that will usually rebalance as you and your body heal) and even illness, as your body rebalances and sheds old ways of existence. It is all part of the process. *Love yourself through it.* There is light on the other side; beautiful, healthy, empowered light. The 'side effects' will balance out and cease, and you will be as a beautiful butterfly emerging from a chrysalis.

If you really check in, you can tell when your body needs things that are easier to digest such as fruit and vegetable juices or when you are in need of a delicious steak or strawberry shortcake or the most decadent and rich chocolate cake you could imagine. EAT IT!!!

This beating up of yourself for what you are wanting and needing and believing you are wrong and that your body is wrong... is it making you happy? Does it have you feeling good about yourself and your life?

What if you and your body are absolutely right??????? How might you feel and live then????? I challenge you to find out what might happen if you begin trusting yourself and your body. Miracles, My Love. Freakin' miracles! They might take some time and wouldn't that be worth it????!!

Small suggestion/aside here: Drinking juices which are 100% pure with no added stuff or sugars; perhaps even juiced by YOU! In your own home and consumed within 24 hours for maximum nutrient benefit. I know this seems specific and nitpicky. I'm only suggesting what might be best in a "My body is craving and needing a break and to slow down. I need to be in 'Rejuvenation mode' right now." way. You can create some really awesome juice blends. Some of my favorites are grapefruit and pineapple or beet, celery, carrot, and apple. Parsley and cucumber is also delicious and very refreshing, juiced.

When eating and purchasing meat, find organic grassfed and/or pasture raised. It may be more expensive. Pesticides, however, are often held in fat. If the animal is eating food with pesticides on or in it, well... Also, we rather overdo corn in our country and I know I personally begin to feel achy and run down when I have too much of it. Beef cattle are often 'finished off' on a corn diet.

I'd invite you to simply take a moment to breathe and check in with your body and how it is feeling and what it is desiring or needing. Even ask, if you feel that might help. Your body will answer you. What sensations are you experiencing? Where are they? Are you envisioning a certain food? Tasting or smelling it? Are you salivating????? Good clues here!!!

This process may take a while as we are not used to doing this and also if we've been consuming a diet rich in processed foods or excessive fruit or other sugars, we may only notice the sugar we are craving. Try to 'look and feel' beyond this. It may be your brain that wants the sugar in an addictive sort of manner, in this instance (which isn't always bad...), not your *being*.

Patience is a virtue. Think LONG term health. Every choice you make in each moment of your day is creating your future. Who do you want to be??? How do you want to feel? What do you want your life to look like?

This process will take time, patience, and love. Give these to yourself freely and abundantly. It's beautiful and okay and you deserve it.

Sometimes it takes me days to realize I've been craving a certain food or foods and then I may crave it for weeks. One summer I wanted lemonade, badly, and I had it daily and found fun new ways to make it! Have you ever tried it with some fresh basil? *Highly* recommend.

Balanced hydration, I've discovered within the last two years, is HUGE. The recommended 8 glasses of water a day can be truly harmful to some people. That research was based on a certain body shape and size and well, you may have noticed, we are all different shapes and sizes. There *is* such a thing as over hydration and it has many of the same symptoms of dehydration. Again, I'd invite you to look this up.

This is why it is so crucial for us to check in, listen, and follow what OUR bodies are trying to tell us.

Again, listen, really listen to your body. Is it really thirsty or is it hungry? Often, we do not eat enough because we are told we eat TOO much. This is something else to question...remember the starvation mode? 2000 calorie a day diets might suit some people. *You* may need more. You may need less. The research on calories and gaining weight was not looked at as closely as it could have been. Researchers are people too. We all sometimes need to look harder, further, deeper.

There was a study done in 1950 by a man named Ancel Keys about starvation. This study was huge and brought to light many interesting and disturbing ideas.
Unfortunately, the biggest idea that was gleaned was that when you consume more calories you gain weight....Yes. AND there was SOOOOO much more to this that was not looked at and *you owe it to yourself to look into this. It has much to do with starvation and yo-yo dieting. Starvation*

20

doesn't only look like skin and bones and sunken eyes. It also has frightening symptoms.

Your body wants, needs, and is meant to move. Find ways you, your being, enjoys moving and do this as often as you feel the need or desire. Attending the local gym or running five miles a day is not necessarily right for you and your body; *especially if you do not enjoy these things.*

Again, learning to read your body's cues i.e. are you feeling antsy and restless or very sluggish? Perhaps these symptoms mean you need to get up and move. If you feel better upon moving, you probably needed that and I'd invite you to keep up with the moving as long as it feels good. If you feel better after moving, great! If not, perhaps you need a rest or a nap. It is possible something deeper is going on. You could try checking in with you again; feel in your body where the uncomfortable feelings are and once you've located them stay with them, they will tell you what you need to know.

Perhaps you are needing to write or sing or chat. Maybe you need to breathe and soothe yourself with a hug or by rubbing your feet or sore spots.

There may not be a need to exercise excessively to lose weight or stay in shape. This has very little to do with losing weight for real or for good and almost everything to do with self-punishment. The exercise you most need is that which lights you up and has you feeling good inside and out. Move your body for the pure enjoyment or desire to move. We are spirit having a human experience. Our body is our vehicle and compass in this life; it is a magnificent creation and moving it for pure enjoyment can be, bliss.

Moving also aids in releasing any negativity we may be harboring. I enjoy doing Tai Chi, yoga, bike riding, hiking on the trails at my favorite park and other new(to me) beautiful outdoor spaces. (Later on we'll learn there is deeper meaning to all of this.) I also enjoy stretching and just sort of haphazardly moving in any way my body is asking. It feels great to listen to and provide my body with what it is asking for.

There is another word that most always comes up at this point of a discussion and that is "Diets". I'm not going to promote any particular diet. In fact, *I'm not going to promote diets, in any form, at all*. I have found, for myself, following any particular diet for a long period of time can be very harmful to one's health. I've also learned that 'dieting' to lose weight just does not work. What does work is learning to listen to and love yourself and your body and give yourself and your body what you are asking for; what you need. When you can do this, you will find amazing, lasting, results.

This journey to learn to love and listen to yourself takes amazing amounts of courage and is the most fulfilling adventure you could ever embark upon. I know this from personal experience.

Your body needs rest. Rest can mean a few moments (or several) of quiet breathing and meditation and *at least* 8 hours of sleep a night. Again, you need to listen to yourself and your body. If 8 hours isn't enough, figure out what is, and provide it for yourself. This will most likely fluctuate.

We do not realize the extreme need for sleep because we can still 'function' if we don't get enough, but our bodies, minds, and spirits know. So many necessary healing and rejuvenating things happen during sleep, that if we want a long meaningful, fulfilling life we cannot afford NOT to get sufficient rest.

Did you know the only time children grow is while they are sleeping? Sleep allows us to heal and to integrate things that happened and were learned during our day. We as people 'grow' while we sleep as well. Sleep allows us and to feel real, happy, and alive. When we get sufficient rest and sleep we are able to thrive and flourish in our life, not just survive.

Don't the words 'flourish' and 'thrive' sound thrilling and more inviting than 'survive'? What might your life look like if you were flourishing? Thriving? Perhaps you'd like to take some time to ponder this and journal about it right now...it could prove to be an incredibly powerful and

23

magical exercise.

Our bodies need to be cleansed properly. It is not necessary to use loads of soap to clean our bodies as it dries out our skin and causes our largest organ of protection to have small cuts which break down the barrier between us and unpleasant germs. This can also happen when we use really hot bath water, which makes me sad because I love hot baths in the winter time and on extra stressful days. I choose to do it anyway though. It is more important to me to rid my being of the stress.

You also want to make sure the soap you are using is safe; meaning, very basically, that it contains only ingredients you can pronounce and which occur in nature, unaltered. Some suggestions are, oatmeal, goat's milk, lavender, coconut oil soap. Almost anything else, even those which claim they are natural (100%, 70%, or otherwise) are toxic and DO cause disease such as cancer.

The thing to note here is that the cleansing formula *has* caused disease or unpleasantness of some sort, just not frequently or severely enough for the government to decide to *inform* you and thus *protect* you and your family by keeping it off of store shelves. Ask yourself this...Do you REALLY want to use ANYTHING that has been known to cause cancer on yourself or your loved ones? Do you really want to take that risk?

This includes laundry, dish, and any other cleaning products. I HIGHLY recommend educating yourself about the dangers of cleaning and beauty products (and that VERY MUCH includes deodorizers! Did you know Febreeze has some 80 different ingredients, some of which are highly dangerous and toxic??? And then, it only MASKS odors!! Essential oils and some water in a spray bottle would ELIMINATE the odors AND put healing and/or calming properties into your air.). Learn to read, and check, labels carefully prior to purchase. 'All Natural' does not mean it is healthy or safe. There are some dangerous things in the world that occur 'naturally'. And there are loop holes which are used to be able to use this label on a product so it will sell.

Our next topic is also 'touchy' and, I feel, needs to be addressed; Vaccines. We seem to be far too scared to discuss this topic. This is understandable. It effects our lives and the lives of our children. AND if it is NOT discussed, it remains a scary, highly charged, topic.

Vaccines started off as an answer to what seemed a serious issue and the theory seems simple enough. The problem, however, is that there was not, nor is there still, enough research done which tested/s the immediate and long term effects or the methods used to give or make the vaccines safe or truly effective. There is just a general, and very serious, lack, covering up, and manipulation of research surrounding this very important and heated

25

topic and you owe it to yourself and your family to find real data from all sides of this issue.

When I began looking for real answers I found *a lot* of information and I will share some general information with you here.

1) Vaccines do not work in our systems the way our systems were meant to handle disease and so have great potential to cause very lasting, long term side effects.

2) Vaccines were introduced right around the same time people were beginning to have access to better nutrition and it is likely, given that our bodies were magnificently and beautifully created to heal themselves, that *this, and not the vaccines,* was the *real* reason diseases began declining.

3) In areas where there have been epidemics, many of the places that received vaccines, experienced actual death from the disease they were aiming to prevent due to lowered immune function from the vaccines and the 'extras' the vaccines contain to 'make them work' in our bodies. Other areas that did not have access to vaccines and contracted the disease di not experience death.

4) The actual diseases the vaccines are meant to prevent are truly only deadly or very harmful to those whose immune systems are already compromised and even in these cases better care and nutrition would be more beneficial than further

26

compromising the immune systems of these people WITH vaccines.

5) Vaccines have to have extra ingredients added to them such as cells from other animals, embryos, etc. in order for our bodies to utilize them. These 'extras' have great ability to cause us further, and long term, harm and to not really protect us from the disease they are meant to anyway.

6) Vaccines are generally only effective for five years. Yep. Five.

This is a big, and often, scary subject, and I invite you to seek answers for yourself until the answers you find give you real peace. There are so many ways to take care of your body, your whole being, that support your overall health, not diminish it, and protect and/or cure you faster and better in the long run. Prevention with supplements and a healthy whole lifestyle, or even contracting the illness and using natural remedies to boost immunity, heal faster and more fully, and ease discomfort are so much healthier and more beneficial for you and your loved ones. It is how you were created, to heal, and stay, in health.

You can find a list of reliable resources at the end of this book.

Another very important and fascinating aspect of our physical health that is important for us to know is about immunity.

It is important to understand something very amazing and very basic...

Our bodies were created to be able to exist healthfully *within* our environment, not be in constant battle with it. *The earth is our home, not our enemy.* Our bodies were created to be able to protect and heal themselves. We were given this amazing power and gift called *Immunity*.

We have immunity that has been with us from our very beginning as an infant and also that was passed to us from our mother in the birth canal (Yes, the birth canal. So when a cesarean section is performed, babies miss out on this valuable gift of immunity from their mothers. Sometimes c-sections are necessary. Most of the time they are not.) We have immunity we gain from existing within, and being exposed to, our environment. This means that if we are otherwise in ultimate health we are able to withstand disease and if we should contract an illness our bodies will fight it and even our symptoms will be almost nothing, if at all.

For example, dreaded Polio. The bacteria which cause Polio exist in the ground, the dirt, where people used to spend much of their time gardening and farming. People often would be exposed to and contract Polio without even necessarily knowing they had it. They might get a

28

fever and feel run down for a few days. As we became weaker and weaker due to poor nutrition and lifestyle our bodies were not as able to fight the infection. For those whose bodies were already most compromised, this meant more obvious symptoms.

The actual number of people who experienced Polio at this level, or worse, paralysis or death, was very small, but numbers and data can be manipulated... Thus a great scare was created and there were these ready-made 'miracle' vaccines to 'protect' us....

One thing that was unknown, or not shared, at the time is that the extra ingredients in the vaccines which made it possible for a body to accept the vaccine compromised the body's immunity in a great way and often paved the way for the disease to spread more quickly and to be more devastating to those it managed to infect, whose systems were already compromised.

This also, then paved the way for other 'side effects' to occur, many of them life-long.

So. By trying to tell the body we had something it needed, which it truly did not, we created a monster mess and cross generational anxiety and insanity... (The definition of insanity is doing the same thing over and over with the same results...)only our *results* keep getting more and more detrimental to our long term health.

Nourish Your Mind

~With Peace

Meditation. This is certainly a buzz word lately. It can be scary because it means being quiet with yourself. And for many of us, this is no small task.

We often equate meditation with sitting cross legged, hands on knees, fingers touching and chanting 'OM' over and over. But. This does not have to be so.

Meditation needs to be done in the way that best suits *you*. I am a Work-at-Home Mama of four. I also homeschool. Time to myself is precious and limited, so my meditation time mostly happens in small bursts of time throughout my day as I'm going about my day. For instance, when I'm washing the dishes (Yes, by hand.) and my mind wanders and an epiphany all of a sudden comes to me or I actually stop stressing over certain things long enough to notice how the water in the sink feels on my hands and how beautiful the soap bubble rainbows look in the morning sunshine. Or how beautiful the birds sound and the rustle of the wind in the trees and the breeze on my skin and through my hair feels. Or the smell of autumn approaching on the evening air. Or when I daydream about my dreams and how it will feel to have them fulfilled.

Yes. All of this is meditation. You are being present with yourself and the earth and spirit, and breathing. Simply taking a pause in your day to take some deep cell/soul cleansing breaths is meditation.

There are times when I will have a rather longish block of time to myself, and at those times I do put on meditative soul stirring music, light candles, equip myself with my journal, tarot and oracle cards, and sit in front of my alter and get present with my breath. At these times, I make a conscious effort to pay attention to my inhalation and exhalation. I have found, my guides know I have limited time so they appear and connect with me quickly, strongly, and deeply. This works because I allow, and am open to, their 'visit' and messages.

You get to find what works for you. It may take some time or no time at all and will most likely change over time, as you do. I recommend patience...with yourself and your guides. Ask them and your angels, guardians, ancestors, totems whomever you speak and connect with, to help you find what you need... *Answers will come.*

Your mind also needs you to be cleared and cleansed of negative words and messages and past stories and beliefs. This is a life-long task. Rather like cleaning your house regularly and during those grand cleaning times in the spring or before a big event.

You see, *what you think; you create*.

31

So, when you perpetually think you are not enough and could do better, that will perpetually be your reality. When you can recognize how amazing and capable you are; you will be.

Ultimately, you must uncover your deep beliefs about yourself and the world you live in. Once you uncover these, if need be, they can be healed, and then you can train your mind to look for a new reality.

An easy and great place to start your search to uncover these deeply held beliefs is in your physical symptoms and feelings that arise. They hold many clues as to the state of your current belief system. Until this belief system is changed, your world will not be able to change.

So, for instance, I have issues with allergies. I have discovered they are a lot about irritation and this is ultimately about what a person is tolerating in life. I now know when my allergies act up it is time for me to stop and check in with myself about what it is I believe I have to be putting up with, that really I don't.

Really what I need to do is love myself and create a boundary around this thing or person I'm tolerating to the point where it no longer irritates me. Sometimes this means getting some perspective so I can change the way *I* see a situation. Sometimes it means saying 'no', this does not work for me and *this* is how it is going to be for me now. I have had to do a lot of work around this in my parenting especially in this last year. It has been hard and messy and amazing and inspiring all at the same time. Beautiful and miraculous things have occurred. It is also ever a work in progress.

Physical symptoms and feelings are our body's way of saying, 'Hey! There is something out of balance here and in order to regain balance, you've gotta pay attention and acknowledge me!' Simply recognizing that you are feeling something, bringing awareness to it, helps the healing process begin.

So, say your shoulders are hurting…you could ask yourself 'What is it I am shouldering right now?' This is also a form of meditation as you need to allow yourself to *Be Quiet* to allow the answers to come.

There are many other ways to sort through your physical symptoms to get to the heart of what is happening with you and heal. Once you get to the core, and you may need assistance, your physical issues will begin to heal. It is even possible for them to disappear instantly.

You are a spiritual being having a human experience here on this plane called Earth. In order to experience humanity, you need a body. Your body and feelings help you navigate this world, they are your compass; along with your spiritual self, your soul.

There is a wonderful book and tool called <u>You Can Heal Your Life</u> by Louise L. Hay. Ms. Hay created a fabulous glossary of physical issues in which she has pinpointed specific emotional issues. She then created affirmations to say to yourself, to your mind, body, and spirit, and to the Universe to begin your healing process. *The trick is, you must hold these beliefs about yourself first and in order to hold these more positive beliefs about yourself, you need to uncover the ones which are keeping you stuck and/or causing issues.* *Awareness is HUGE and most of our beliefs are subconscious.*

Ultimately, our greatest, and most simple issues, are with loving and approving of ourselves. This is absolutely at the core of our life's issues.

There is deep work to be done here and there are amazing coaches and others in the world who can help with this work. It is truly magical. I have personally experienced it. Please see the 'resources' section for some fabulous suggestions. In my work as a coach, I assist my clients to get to the heart of their physical issues and it is amazing to see the results in their lives!

So. In every moment, in your mind, and in your actions, *you* are creating your reality...

What do you want your reality to be? Who do you want to be?

Often it does not appear to be so simple to recreate our reality and heal. We feel stuck, blocked, and even just shut down. We may feel anger or even just numb.

This is all normal and okay. We are human and imperfect, and beautiful and perfect all at the same time. Life is a journey and journeys include hills, mountains, valleys, plains, waterfalls, calm peaceful paths, jagged rocky caverns, streams, swirling whirling rapids; all kinds of terrain, as do our lives. The secret is in how you choose to view and react to life. It is very possible to hold beliefs within your being we may be unaware of. These unconscious beliefs can keep us reacting and viewing life in the same way, to the same stimuli, repeatedly.

When this happens, you may get to a point where you've had enough. Your life just feels as though it is not working and everything you try doesn't seem to help, or at least not completely.

Sometimes this means there is deeper work to be done. Other times this means you need to step back and gain some perspective or simply employ some patience and quiet until you can see an opening. Sometimes from this space, you'll have an 'Aha!' moment.

This may feel bad, but there truly is no good or bad in life. We as humans place judgment. *The Universe does not know judgment; only how to create the way for us to live the life we imagine.*

The Universe also does not measure time as we do. It may be that we are stuck, blocked, or exhausted for what seems like an eternity to us. We may feel anger around this and this is okay and will need to be felt fully to be cleared. After this has been accomplished though, and you are still waiting, what do you choose to do with your waiting time? Grumble it away or live it joyfully? It is okay to still enjoy life while waiting...it is recommended in fact, as it tends to bring what you desire faster. It is certainly more fun and life is meant to have us feeling good!

I'm not saying I've perfected ANY of this or that I always choose joy. I've played the victim for most of my life. It has only been recently that this no longer HAS to be my reality. I've broken my cycle of reacting the same way to the same stimuli repeatedly. It feels FABULOUS to be in this place; to no longer have to be the victim of my own thoughts and beliefs. If this can be my reality; it can also be yours.

Nourish Your Spirit

Our Spirit is our essence. It is who we are at our core. It is God, Goddess, the Universe, the Divine, the Creator, Source; whatever name feels best to you.

Spirit is who we know we are when we are still, quiet, and truly check in with our heart. It is that strength, that quietness you feel smiling and assuring, always. It is your Intuition.

To nourish your spirit you get to allow it to sing, to soar, to be free, to be heard, to speak, to shine. You get to discover what things allow your spirit to express her/himself, and feel most alive.

We are creative Beings. Being creative simply means to bring forth something of yourself. We are, at our core, creative. We are creation. Created. There is no way to NOT be creative. There are some ways we personally allow our spirit to soar and create more than others. This is for us to know and discover on our own by participating in experiences which help us to find our personal likes and dislikes.

Writing, talking, singing, dancing, laughing, serving others are all ways my spirit soars. When I am allowing my spirit to be expressed my mind calms, the endless chatter, helpful and harmful, ceases and my body relaxes and feels ALIVE. When we feel this way, ALIVE, we are SO healthy;

mind, body, spirit. *This* is when a path opens for our metabolism, our fire, to burn its brightest and strongest and we are able to easily be in ultimate health.

As children, if allowed, our spirits soared effortlessly and endlessly. Sometimes our spirits were shut down very early on by the adults or caregivers in our lives and their own fears. Many of us have allowed society to succeed in shutting down our spirits as we grew into adulthood.

In order to regain our balance, our health of mind, body, spirit, we must reclaim and reawaken our spirits and have the courage to allow them to be expressed.

So? Where to start? How to begin?

Getting out in nature, (remember earlier when I was talking about exercise and said getting outside would come up later….here it is!!) with our Mother is always an excellent way to reconnect and reawaken our spirit. When we step outside, even doing something simple such as sitting on the ground and feeling the earth beneath our body, or watch the trees as they sway in the wind, and just simply BE, we get back into our bodies and connect with our spirit and Source.

There will begin to be a stirring in our bodies, in our solar plexus and our heart which tells us, 'You are alive.' You may want to close your eyes to feel this more fully and you may begin to smile, to feel more at peace and connected. Once you have reveled in this feeling, you may want to move on to discover what it is your heart wants you to know or remember. Ask your heart, 'What do you want me to know in this moment?' A vision may appear in your mind or you may sense a feeling, an awareness, about you.

Listen.

Quietly.

Allow your heart to speak to you.

From here you will begin to learn what it is that lights you up; what it is that makes your heart sing!

For women especially, (and men, this is important to know) it is important to note that in our society we are very often expected to be contrary to who and what we are. *We embody the feminine essence which is without bounds and longs to express and create and to simply BE.*

The feminine essence needs to be able to be expressed and lived. One of the reasons we have such horrible issues with our feminine parts and processes and functions is because we ignore, neglect, and outright refuse and/or downplay these parts of ourselves. These issues exist because our beings are crying out to be heard, acknowledged, loved, and honored.

One way women used to honor themselves and their cycle (which actually used to literally follow the moon cycles because of the honoring of the way of life; nature. And yes, it IS possibly to get back on that cycle…) was to gather together during their 'Moon Time', or period, in a tent to bleed, rest, create, and just be women. Women in a tribe would all bleed at the same time (full moon) each month. This time was considered sacred and honored.

You could greatly improve any unpleasant PMS symptoms or other feminine 'issues' by honoring this time for yourself each month. You probably have days, during this time, where you are more tired, especially the first few days. On these days, or at least one, could you take the day(s) for yourself to rest, be quiet, do gentler activities, take a bath, journal, create? I invite you to try it for several months and see what things might change in your life. Your bleeding time is not a curse. It is a beautiful gift. It is a time to shed what no longer serves you and to take beautiful time for yourself, to fill you back up, so that you can beautifully return to your life and families and other loved ones and care for them from this place of abundance. *How might your life look differently?*

Men, making space to allow for the women in your life to honor this for themselves is a beautiful and perfect way to provide for them. AND, you have aspects of the feminine within you. *How can you honor this for them, for yourself? How can you make sure you are living your life from a space of being cared for, creative, nurtured? How can you create this for yourself? How might YOUR life look differently if you did this?*

Another way to go about learning what makes your spirit soar is to remember your childhood. As a child, what did you love? What did you enjoy and get lost spending time doing? Does that, or some form of it, still light you up now?

What do you find yourself daydreaming about? What makes your heart skip a beat or race? What makes you smile, brings tears to your eyes, or makes you feel as though you'd like to scream to the world, 'This is AMAZING!!!'?

Begin to say, 'Yes' to opportunities which present themselves, even if at first they do not really interest you. If you don't try, you'll never know. You may discover the love of your life...

Nourish Your Soul

I believe our Soul is separate from our Spirit in that it has a purpose or mission on this Earth. We are a spiritual being that is a soul. Our soul lives forever and makes a choice to have this earthly human experience.

The situation we are born into depends on what our soul chooses as our purpose for this life. As a soul, we spend our human lifetime discovering and fulfilling our purpose and finding 'Home' within ourselves.

Our soul comes to this earthly plane with a mission, a purpose, a destiny to fulfill, a path to follow. Our *spirit* and our body are our guides on this path; along with any other guides we may ask for assistance. They help us to know if we are on the right path. When our spirit feels dead, and we are depressed, in continuous pain, have unhealthy bodies and minds, it is then we know we are not following our path. (This can also show up in our toes! :) And you can contact me at www.jessicalalden.com for a toe reading. ;)) This can cause us to feel intense emotions, and our bodies to feel intense sensations.

When these emotions, sensations, continue on for a prolonged period of time (and even before that), it is time to stop and ask, 'Why?' 'What is happening?' What do I need to do, discover, work with, feel into, to bring about change?'

Remembering...

I believe our soul knows exactly who we are, where we came from, and what our purpose is. It is our humanity which allows the forgetting. I believe it is possible to be still and quiet enough to sense what we know and remember about who we are, to bring it into the light.

I've created and experienced, for myself, several meditations where I've delved deeply into the dark of my soul and brought answers into the light. It can be done.

I believe also that, as humans, we are not meant to exist, BE, travel, alone and that many spectacular tools have been placed, and exist, within our reach if only we ask and search. Our humanity is just as beautiful and precious as our spirituality. *Humannness is no fault or sin to overcome.* It just is. It is perfect. It is a way to exist, it is a tool in itself and if we need to employ, or desire to employ, tools to help us know and remember, that is perfect as well.

There are many amazing ways to connect with your soul and the Divine. I believe we are all here, on this earth, with any number of spirit guides, totems, and angels, whatever you choose to call them, all of whom are available and happy to help us. We need only ask. There are many ways they communicate with us and us them. Following are some methods I enjoy and have found very useful.

Animals can help us to understand ourselves, our spirit and soul. You might notice a certain animal keeps showing up in your life in various places or situations. You might have a unique encounter with a raccoon and then see it in other interesting or ordinary places or it may come up in conversations, books, movies, in traveling. If an animal

43

seems to be 'visiting' you, it may be time to ask what message they have for you. You can find out more information by doing a simple web search for 'raccoon symbolism' or 'medicine'. Each animal has its own unique 'medicine' or message to share, teach, and help us learn.

Oracle and tarot cards are also an excellent tool for connecting with the Divine, our angels, guides or totems. Using a pendulum, meditating, and paying attention to our dreams are equally useful and fun. Meditating, to glean answers from within YOURSELF is about as amazing, precious, and perfect as it gets.

You could have your palm or toes read or even have a tarot/oracle card reading done for you.

There are so many ways to work with your guides, those who walk this life with you 'unseen' , to know if you are on your path. These are simply a few suggestions, ways I employ, trust, and enjoy. I invite you to try them, and find others that light you up.

Find what feels right and good to you. You are meant to feel joy and follow your joy through this life.

This is YOUR life; YOUR body, YOUR mind, YOUR spirit, YOUR soul. YOU get to fine tune EVERYTHING in your life to what feels right and good to YOU. Your body, feelings, heart are all compasses to help you create the life that is just right for YOU. All you need do is be quiet and listen and then DO. Sometimes 'DO' means wait and be patient. Sometimes 'DO' means rest and be quiet and still. Sometimes 'DO' means go run a marathon or around the block. Sometimes 'DO' means clean your space and declutter. Sometimes 'DO' means spend time daydreaming about what it is you want. 'DO' is a lot of things. Above all 'DO' is what your heart and body are asking you to do. When you listen, you will be in alignment with WHO you are and your metabolism, health, life will flourish.

Wishing you bliss!

45

This writing, this work, started out as a way for me to explain good, sound, *simple* nutrition, and turned into a sharing of the truth of my heart and my life to date. There is more, so much more…Life is not meant to be a constant struggle. It can be simple and easy and is truly meant to be enjoyed.

This is simply an introductory guide, and hopefully a new perspective, for you to begin considering.

There are so many more specific ideas and tools, modes of healing, etc. to share. Each of them has books and volumes of information on their own. You get to follow your own heart to find what most speaks to you at any given moment in your life.

Wishing you exquisite peace, love, and joy!!!

If you are interested to know more, or would love help along your journey, I am here to listen to, and hear, your story. I will hold space for you to glean what it is you truly desire in your life, and then work with you as you begin to travel your unique path to attain that which your heart desires. Thank you for allowing me to share with you. I wish you Peace and Joy on your beautiful journey.

You can contact me at www.JessicaSutter.com or jessicasutterconnect.com

Namaste,

Jessica Sutter

Resources

www.180degreehealth.com ~ Matt Stone

You Can Heal Your Life by Louise L. Hay

www.angeltherapy.com ~Doreen Virtue

http://tenpennyimc.com/ and type in 'vaccines' in the search box.

https://www.facebook.com/notes/dr-tenpenny-on-vaccines/new-rules/363686858343

http://www.nvic.org/

http://www.nccn.net/~wwithin/homeo.htm

http://pathwaystofamilywellness.org/

www.JessicaSutter.com

www.visionarymom.com

www.theorganicsister.com

www.leoniedawson.com

www.intouchinlife.com

There are so many, many more resources.
These are a great place to start... :)